Contents

Dedication

This book is dedicated to Alley Daley

And

My great, great grandmother

Emma Armitage

And

Those still waiting for answers

Preface

Some people live with chronic pain for most of their lives and never find an answer for the apparently unrelated symptoms which continue to dog them and disrupt their lives. They never do manage to piece together all the bits of the missing jigsaw and live with the consequences of that for the rest of their lives.

The impact of chronic pain is far reaching. It affects relationships which often break down leaving families reeling from the shock.

Finances are another casualty of an individual living with chronic pain. It often leaves people unable to work at all. Pain can be all consuming and, sometimes, there are not adequate remedies.

The cost of disability is high. It is far higher than the pittance given out by government for which individuals have to repeatedly account. We need a name putting to our pain to give it credibility but often we are denied this. Medical science has still a long way to go but so often if there is not an answer to be found in a text book then the existence of your pain is denied. At best it will be labelled as a manifestation of mental illness.

There is no doubt that chronic pain can lead you down the path of depression and anxiety but these symptoms did not come first. They are the consequence of an as yet unidentified, but very real - medical condition.

Physical pain is difficult enough to deal with but it becomes an unbearable cross when faced with the disbelief of people – many of them in the caring professions – whose own helplessness at being able to diagnose a condition results in them taking a step back from the patient, leaving the patient even more isolated than they already were.

It is good to acknowledge the pain even if an answer cannot be provided. It is good for the medical profession to acknowledge that they don't have the answers to everything, but that they accept that the pain still exists. That's when the patient breathes a small sigh of relief and feels able to continue the journey with the person who is caring for them.

Along my own journey with chronic pain, I have been accused of exaggerating the hurt and the discomfort. The form these insults take are often in line with current government thinking on the 'disabled' in society. We are viewed negatively and it is not even subtle. We are made to feel guilty for being born with a condition we did not want in the first place. My pain started when I was a child before the time of DLA and PIP before I knew what a 'benefit' was for.

I was never rewarded for being ill. It was just a nuisance that had to be got over as quickly as possible. As I got older its impact on my life is probably better not being dwelt upon. It would be just another insult to the injury already suffered.

I have friends who are chronically ill. They have been labelled lazy or 'swinging the lead' etc. My friend who was labelled with the latter was told he was fit for work by somebody who was supposed to be competent enough to undertake an assessment. It would not take a lot to understand that the hollow cheeks and ashen colour were signs of someone who was very ill

Only days later after being told he was fit for work, my friend was admitted to hospital and spent seven weeks there undergoing two major operations which were necessary as a result of the damage his undiagnosed Crohn's disease had done. A couple of years later he still has a suprapubic catheter in. It is unlikely he will ever be fit for work.

This book is about my chronic pain. It became my companion when I was a child and it has accompanied me ever since. I did not know its name. I only knew it as a charlatan, a thief, who took what little I had and then went only to return disguised as something else – slippery customer it was - to steal yet another portion of my life.

I have spent a large part of my life waiting in cold and impersonal hospital corridors, hoping against hope that this swindler would be identified. It never was until recently, but along the way I was gathering pieces of a jigsaw - although I did not know it at the time – which helped me piece together what was happening and to eventually identify this crook.

I came across this recently

If you can't connect the issues think connective tissues

 I wish that I had come across it many years ago.

The Beginning

I have always been in pain. As far as I can remember I have been enveloped in a diffuse sea of pain which sometimes breaks out with a roar, frustratingly limiting what I can do and preventing me from sleeping. It affects my mood and my ability to think. It affects every part of me and, as such, it affects those around me.

I have always been aware of my pain but I have not closely examined it. It became a part of me - my unwanted traveling companion which, no matter how I tried, I could not shake off.

It is not emotional pain although I can see why some people might think that it was. Life has been, by no stretch of the imagination, easy. It has really been one hard slog. It is not easy being abused – both physically and mentally - as a child or bringing up three children on the autistic spectrum. Everything impacts on your relationships. Everything!

It is hard enough dealing with the pain, never mind supporting others who cannot see what I am dealing with. Others, who think that their needs should always come first and are blind to the burden I carry every day. I do not have a personality which jumps up and down – not verbally anyway – and insists on getting people's attention. I was brought up to be quiet and well mannered. When faced with a chameleon of an illness, such personality traits can prove to be your downfall.

It took me a long time not to accept the professional opinions of experts. Their opinions on my pain did not negate it. It was real enough.

To begin with, as a child, the joints in my hand, particularly my thumb, became very sore. I was prescribed a noxious black ointment which turned olive green when I rubbed it on my skin. It did not relieve the pain. I endured it for many months and then the pain extended to my right shoulder and my legs. It has been my bedfellow ever since.

I was prescribed Butazolidine. I cannot recall if it worked. It was eventually taken off the market anyway because of a rare but serious side effect - that of hepatotoxicity. I became use to leaning my head on one side trying to dislodge the pain. That didn't work either.

Most of the time my brain didn't function either. That was peculiar having an IQ of over 150 and finding that my capacity to think only extended to an hour. I bruised without being able to recall when I had injured myself. I complained – more to myself than anybody else – that I took a long time to heal. I decided I needed more vitamin C. In spite of taking adequate doses it did not help one bit.

We were quite a flexible family. My sister could easily go over into the crab position. My friend could touch her wrist with her thumb on the same side as her wrist. I could also do this but nobody else could. I could also do the splits but then I thought that everybody else must be able to do that anyway. It never entered my head that they wouldn't be able to. My mother could lean over, keep her knees straight and place her palms flat on the ground. It was her party piece.

The migraines dogged my life. I barely existed. Medication only worked for half an hour and the relentless pain would come back and come back and come back.

My jaw kept getting stuck. I could not understand this. It was painful and disabling. In the end I cut up my food into very tiny pieces. L used one hand to feed myself; the other hand I kept pressed firmly to my jaw in an effort to stabilise it. It took months before it was less problematical but, I think, only because I ate only foods which are soft and can be eaten without chewing.

Even today, I have a soft food diet. Chewing is painful but on occasions when I have temporarily forgotten the pain and discomfort, I will try some steak again. The result is always the same. My jaw locks and I have to massage it for a while before it returns to normal. Over succeeding weeks it remains problematical until it settles down again. This is one of the reasons why I do not enjoy going to the dentist. I have to open wide and this sets my jaw off again.

To add to the severe pain which are associated with migraines, I had – and still have - repeated bouts of sinusitis. The pain is horrendous. I bled regularly from my nostrils every time I had sinusitis and still I had three young children to look after and a job to go to.

I had extensive pain in my neck and large muscle on my back. I was referred to physio but they could only address one area of pain. In the end the pain was never addressed – nothing that ever was prescribed took the pain way apart from Vioxx. That was eventually taken off the market because of concerns about its side effects. There wasn't a substitute medication which I could take so continued to live with chronic and intractable pain.

One day I woke up in severe pain with a very swollen ankle. I hadn't had an accident. I went to A&E and saw Dr McKenzie. He was very nice, initially. He asked me how I had injured myself and I stated that I did not know. He did not believe me. His attitude changed. I was quiet then and bewildered by his response. I went home. I had to walk along the edge of the hospital corridor wall in order to have some support. No one stopped and helped. My tears were not external but I was crying on the inside.

On another occasion my foot was so painful that I could not lift it up to place it on the next step of the stairs. I stood on the stairs crying, helpless and wondering why this kept happening to me.

For some reason I became constipated. I could not understand this. I was about twenty five, took lots of exercise and ate lots of fibre. It was intractable. For a while, magnesium sulphate worked and then it ceased to do so. I discussed it with my GP. I was prescribed medication. It helped for a short while and then ceased to do so. I went back to him and informed him that the medication was no longer working. He said that he could give me something stronger but that I would regret it.

I informed him that I would not so he prescribed me this stronger medication and I did not regret it. I have been on this and additional medication ever since. That Is, for forty years.

I sincerely hoped that one day I would be free from taking this medication but now I know I will not.

When I started nursing, I was beset by my 'bad' shoulder again. I frequently went over on my ankles. Sprains and strains were part and parcel of my life. One day when I turned on the tap I sprained my wrist. I could not turn the tap on again for many weeks using my dominant hand and I could not turn it on with my left hand which has little strength and dexterity anyway. I felt helpless and bewildered, angry and frustrated. My features became passive as though the effort of coping with the pain took away my personality.

My mother had some very pronounced varicose veins removed. She also had diverticulitis. I did not know then how important that this information would eventually be. I was handed pieces of a jigsaw bit by bit and did not know it. I was too busy working, bringing up children and coping with intractable pain.

On one particular day when my ankle blew up like a balloon, I was referred to the rheumatology department. By the time my appointment had arrived in the post, that ankle had recovered but the other was now also very swollen and painful. It was thought that this had occurred as I would be putting more weight on my right foot since the tendonitis had occurred in my left ankle. I knew that wasn't the case.

I had developed a malar rash. I took a photo of it convinced that all the pain I was experiencing was due to lupus. I took the photo in and informed the consultant that I had a picture of a malar rash. 'Yes!' She said, 'I am looking at it now.'

When I looked in the mirror I was indeed sporting a very noticeable malar rash.

I did not want lupus but I wanted an explanation. I did not get one; the ANA came back negative. Test for Rheumatoid Factor also came back negative. I became quite paranoid thinking that the medics would think I was making it up. At one physiotherapy appointment one physio informed me that lots of people made things ups as they liked the contact from another person.

I know what I would have liked to have said to her but I was just too polite. Instead I went home and cried. Most of the time other people's touch is actually painful to me so she was off the mark there.

I wish people would think before they speak.

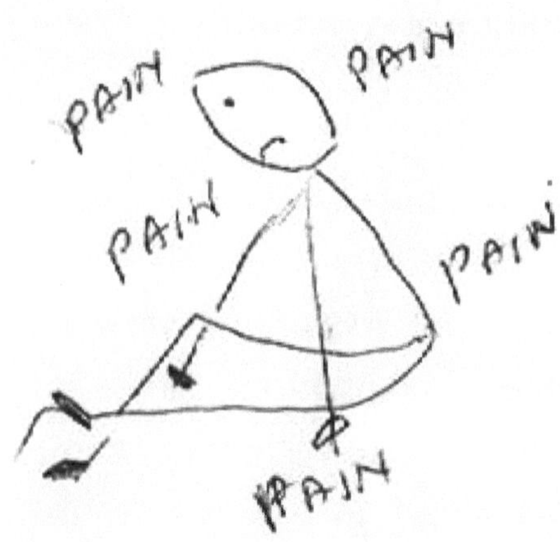

My three children were born easily. Short labours, no stitches. I did not know that this was another of those jigsaw pieces. Hyper elastic skin enables easy births.

Many members of my family have syndactyl. This is webbing of the toes. My joints here are very mobile and can contort themselves into lots of unnatural positions. I did not know that this was a missing piece of the jigsaw.

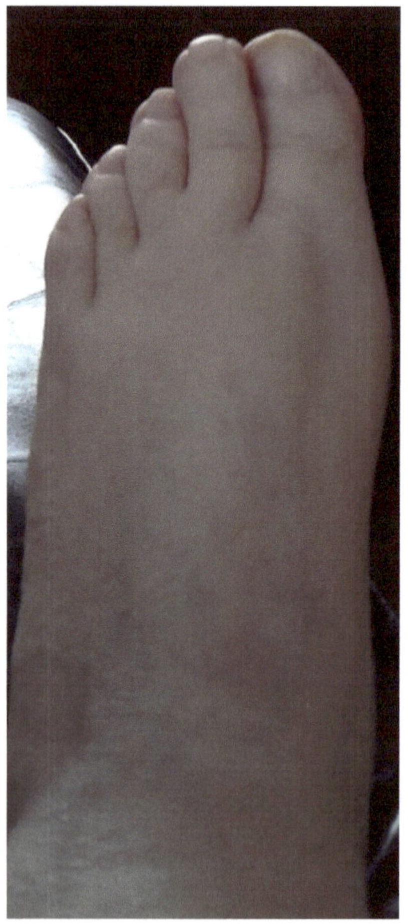

 Syndactyl of second and third toes and visible veins on the foot showing fragility of the skin. Toes, 2, 3 and 4 are hypermobile.

The veins on my hands are very prominent too. The skin is fragile and easily shows the veining beneath it. This was another piece of the jigsaw.

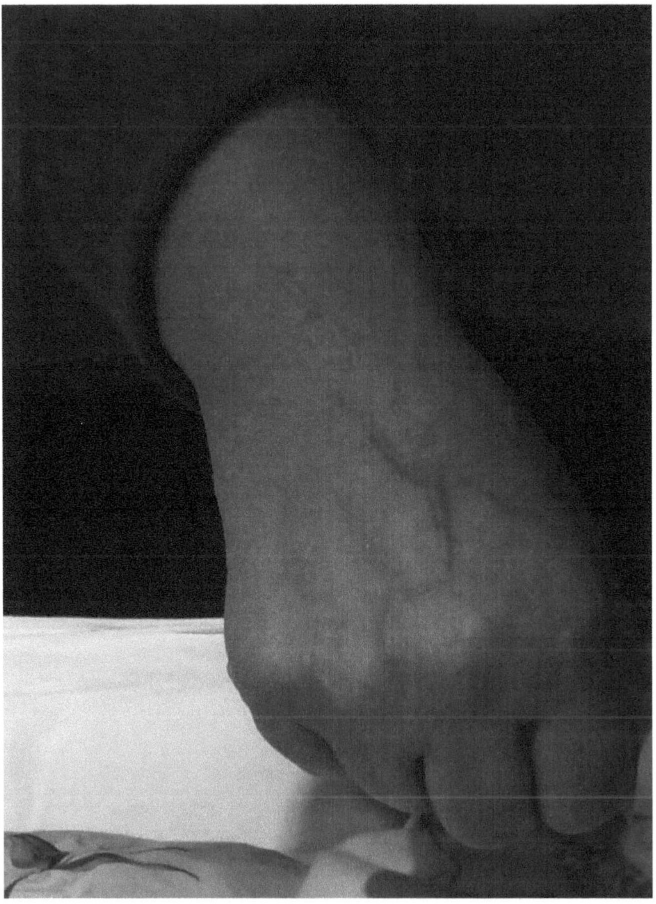

Picture showing veins of the hand due to skin fragility.

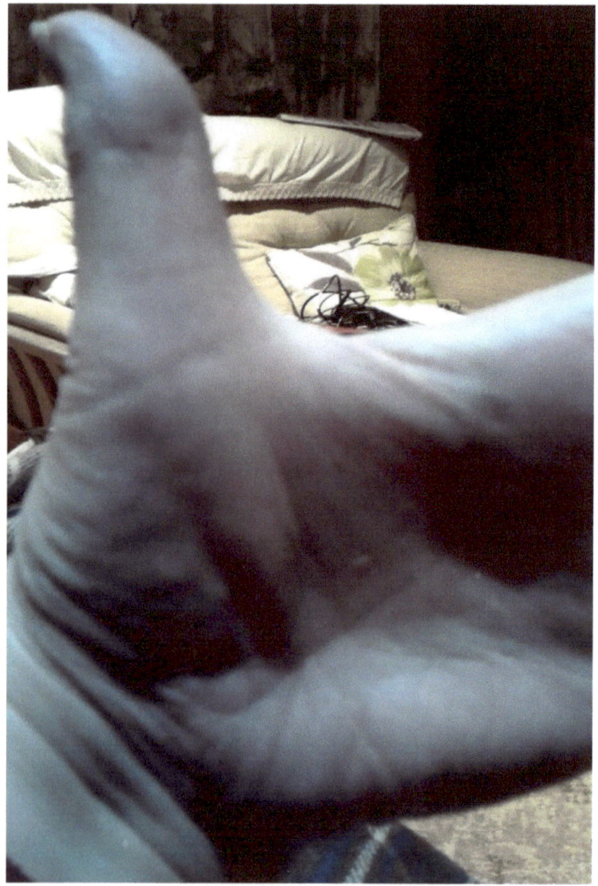

The tissues of my skin are loose.

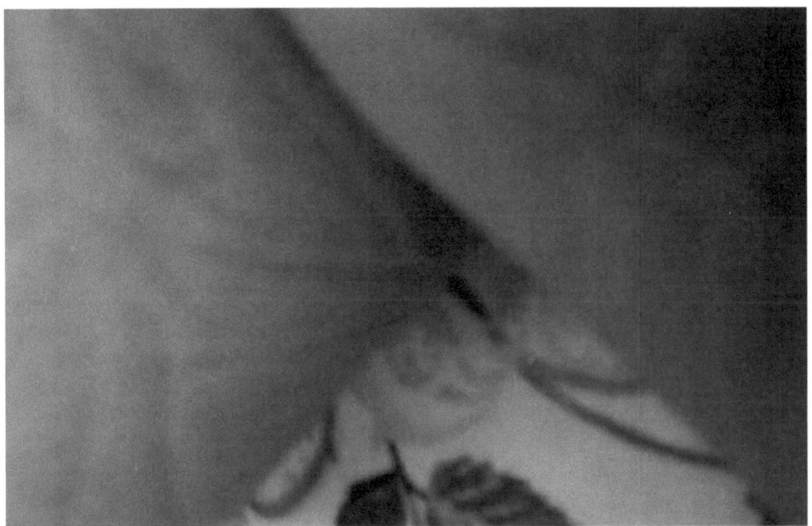

The tissues of my skin are so fragile that clothing is imprinted onto it. This is called dermographics. Most clothing is painful on my skin. I can only wear wool and cotton. Seams are painful and bring me out in sores. The above is the result of wearing cotton cords.

When I press the end of my fingertips, the indentation remains for a long, long time and I have stretchy skin.

When I pull the skin on the back of my hand, it stretches and does not snap back into place when released.

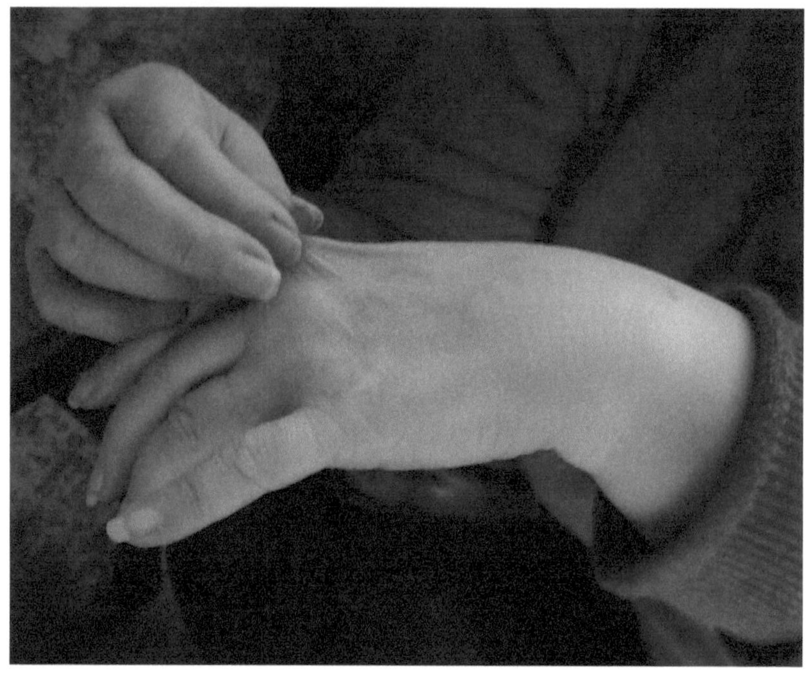

Along with weak ankles, I have hypermobile knees.

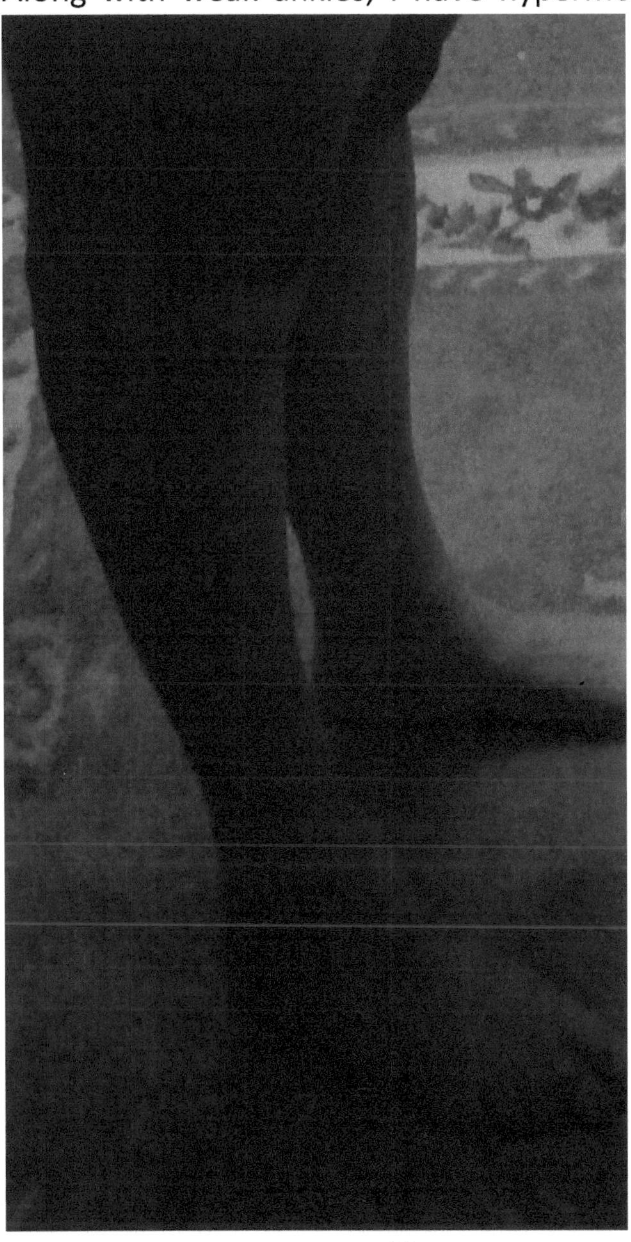

They can bend backwards. They do this when I am walking. It throws me off balance and is also very painful.

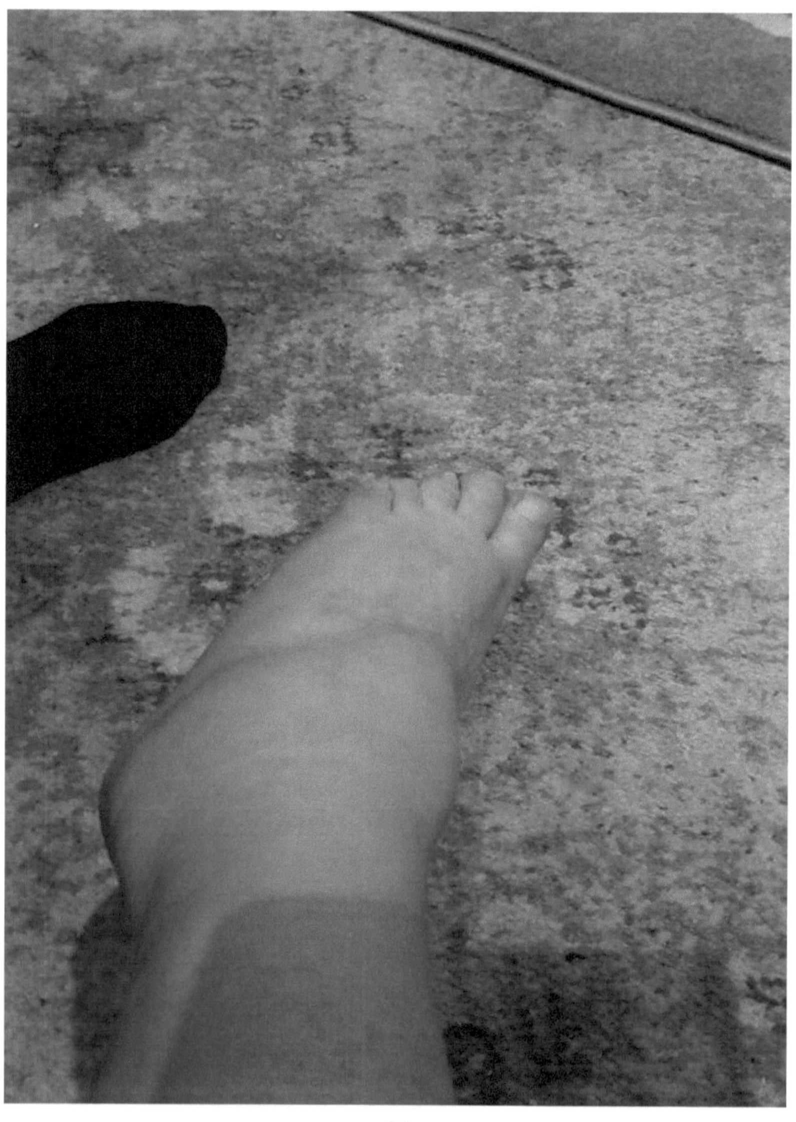

  When my feet swell I cannot wear shoes and my feet become numb as well as painful. I know, it appears to be a contradiction of terms. I have to keep my feet up at all times when I am not walking.

My throat also swells up. I have difficulty swallowing even when my throat isn't swollen.

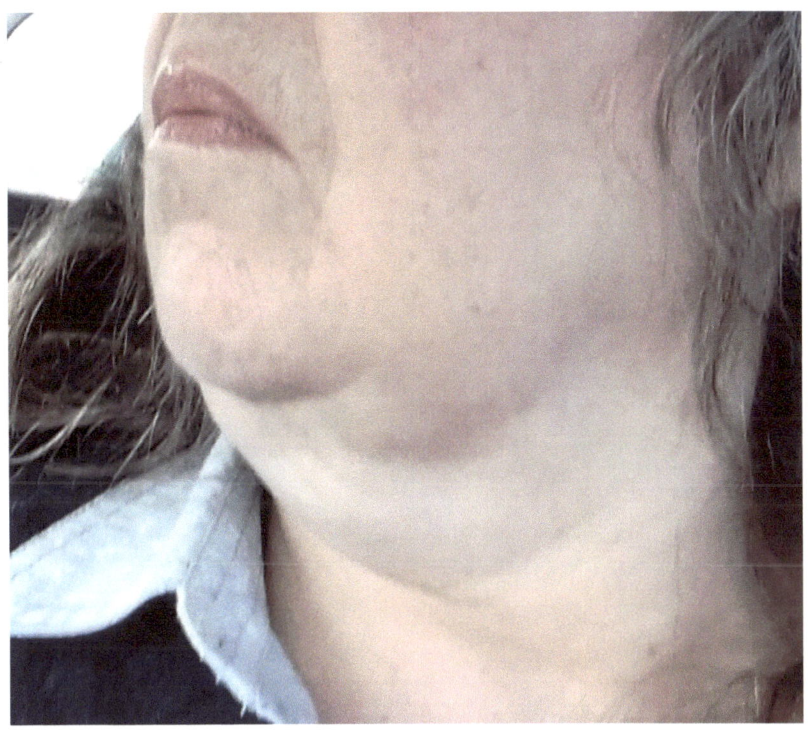

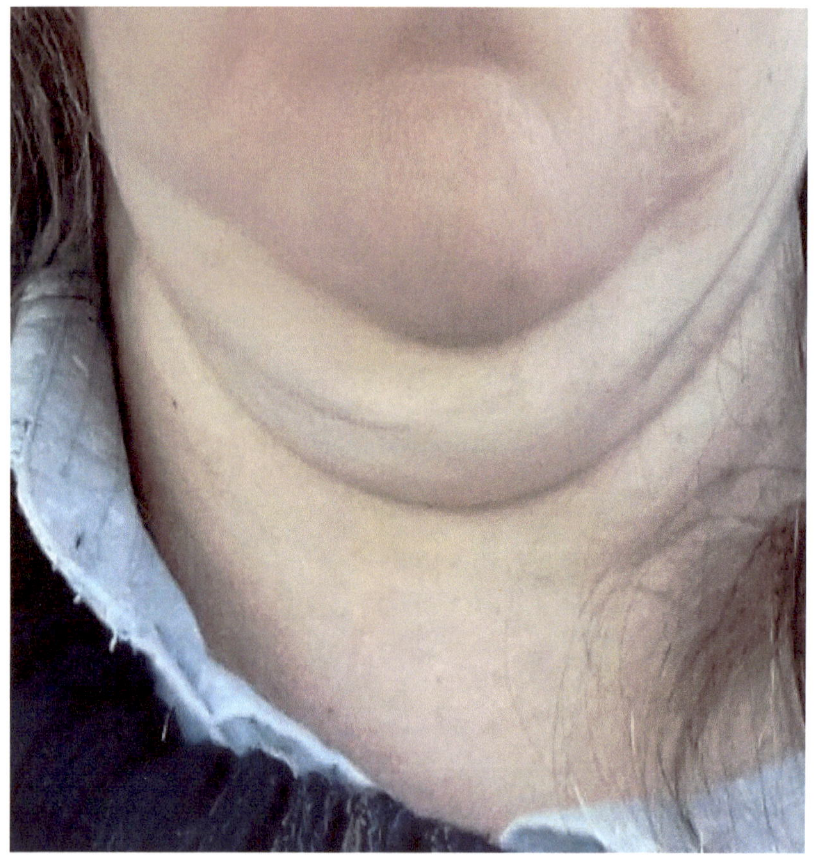

Swelling of throat – note the laxity of tissues.

You need to know what my neck looks like when the tissues aren't swollen.

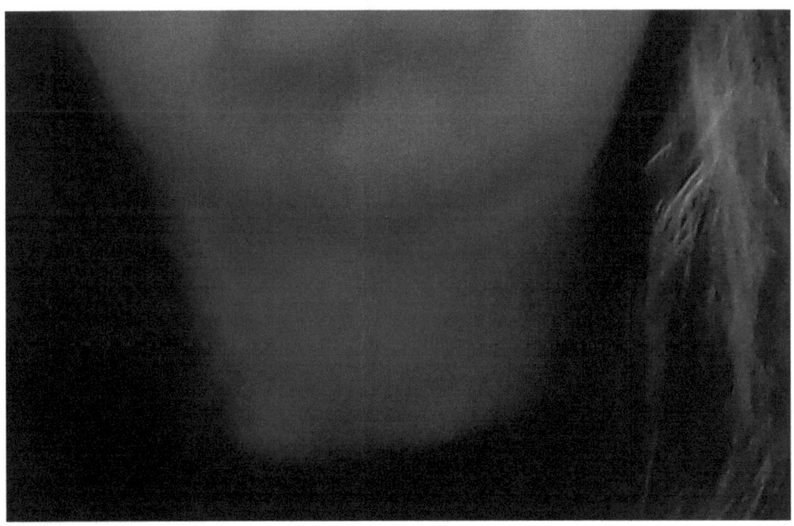

Non swelling of tissues.

There's a big difference isn't there?

I bruise very easily. When I had an operation in September 2016, the anaesthetist said my veins were so fragile that they just broke up as soon as he put the needle in. He attempted a few times to get the needle in both arms to find a vein that he could use.

My arms and the backs of my hands looked a little like this. It was not a good look, I can tell you.

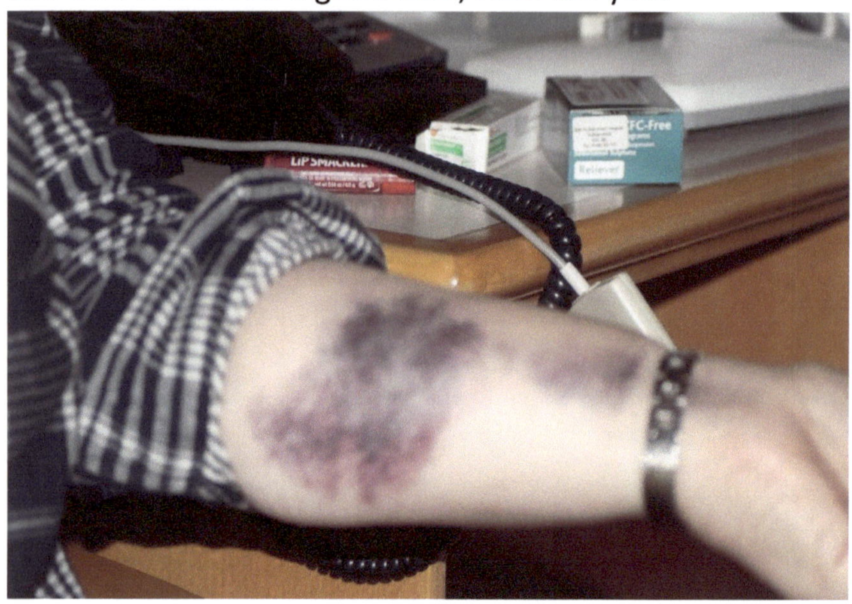

I also had a diastasis recti of five inches. This is a gap between the abdominal walls, which shouldn't be there. This was another missing piece of the jigsaw. When the connective tissue isn't very strong then it can't do its job properly. Hernia type situations are very common in conditions like Ehlers Danlos Syndrome.

FAMILY HISTORY.

A family history is important but with conditions like hypermobility it is easy to not connect the dots up - to not understand there can be a relationship between symptoms which do not appear to be connected to each other.

Symptoms, even within family members with the same condition, can vary widely and this is down to our different genetic arrangement. What has my aunt with thread veins, obesity and arthritis got to do with someone who has dislocated their shoulder, has cigarette scarring and finds food gets stuck in their throat. At first glance there does not appear to be association whatsoever. So, we deny, on this evidence alone, that there is anything which appears to run in our families which could account for our symptoms.

I suppose if I had dislocated my joints a number of times then that might have set alarm bells ringing but this was not the case for me. I have just had constant strains and sprains – with all the pain which this entails - which are hardly given a cursory glance. 'Go home, apply ice, elevate your limb and apply pressure' we are told.

It trips easily off the tongue and meanwhile the years of pain and lost opportunity are ignored.

I had heard of Ehlers Danlos Syndrome, but knew little of it. I was more interested in neuro-degeneration and had completed some research in statins and cognitive decline. I had plenty of time to ponder on this aspect of my research since the pain from my muscles and joints was relentless and kept me awake at night. If I pulled open drawers I more often than not pulled the muscles in my hand. It was painful but it had become the norm for me.

A few months ago a fifth cousin contacted me. She had a daughter called Alice who had Ehlers Danlos Syndrome. It seemed severe. I started researching this syndrome as I always do when faced with a medical condition I know little of. It was like looking at my life really. Every symptom that I had ever had could be encapsulated in this syndrome.

I had undertaken quite a bit of research on the paternal grandmother's father side when I was looking at the genetic pattern of chronic glomerular nephritis which my dad had died from.

I hadn't started on the paternal grandmother's mother's side although I had collected a lot of death certificates. I did have the death certificate of my GG grandmother, Emma Armitage, who was the sister of Hannah who headed my fifth cousin's side of the family.

Emma was just thirty years old when she died of perforation of the stomach. This type of medical accident is found in Ehlers Danlos Syndrome vascular type (vEDS) which leads to fragility of blood vessels, bowel and uterus that leads to spontaneous rupture.

I have very fragile blood vessels but the vascular type of EDS does not generally have stretchy skin and I do have that in some areas.

I do not know that much about Emma's daughter, Ann. She lived to a good age and at the end of her life had dementia.

Ann had a number of children – nine to be exact and most of them had some vascular problem as well as joint pain. My grandmother was said to suffer from arthritis as did her sister. Laurie. My grandma had chronic constipation. I was a child when I found this out. I don't think I was supposed to know but Grandma had to have a mug of slippery elm every night. I was a curious child and asked a relative what it was for. I was told in a hushed whisper that it was to help with Grandma's bowels.

My grandma's older sister, Laurie, died from

1a Cerebral haemorrhage

b Arterial degeneration

2 Rheumatoid arthritis

1a AND 1b are very much related to vEDS and I suspect that the rheumatoid arthritis was very much the joint pain which is part and parcel of the hypermobility of EDS.

One of my grandmother's younger brother – William Arthur -   died aged 25 years from a condition known as abdominal actinmycosis. This is an infection which usually follows a break in the gastrointestinal mucosa. In EDS the intestinal lining is fragile and easily broken and this could afford the opportunity for a bacterial infection to take hold.

MATERNAL SIDE

My mother, who is ninety two, and her two older sisters and two younger sisters are still alive. Their lives have been characterised by arthritic pain. Most of them appear to be on the autistic spectrum. They show lots of traits, anyway. Autistic Spectrum Disorder and hypermobility syndrome are comorbidities, but I cannot say for certain that their arthritic pain is due to EDS.

One of my aunts has suffered from overweight, arthritic pain and very obvious fine red veins on her cheeks. All these signs are connected to EDS. She is now in a wheelchair.

My maternal grandfather was said to have suffered from constant joint pain. Perhaps that is what made him the morose figure he appeared to be.

My mother used to have migraine, bulging varicose veins and joint problems. Her hips and knee joints – apart from one – have been replaced. She has diverticulitis. These conditions are associated with EDS and, of course, my mother used to be able to touch the floor with her palms flat while keeping her knees straight. This is one of the criteria from the Beighton score for EDS.

I do not think that I would have begun to have piece these bits of the jigsaw together so soon if my fifth cousin had not contacted me. That set me off on an interesting and all-consuming path. I love research.

Nearly There

I have had times when I have just 'conked' out. I don't lose consciousness but I go very weak and I am unable to do anything. At such times I am very vulnerable. Most of the time, but not every time, this occurs after I have been eating. This suggests some type of anaphylaxis especially as I have other allergy type symptoms.

With EDS there is a common associated condition known as postural tachycardia syndrome (PoTS). In this condition the autonomic system can be dysregulated and this can be felt as

- Dizzy spells
- Facial flushing
- Palpitations

These symptoms can occur when a change of posture occurs but sometimes, as they do with me, they occur after eating.

Studies have shown that autonomic symptoms and gastrointestinal symptoms are the two areas which impact on the quality of life for those with EDS. These are related to EDS types

- Classical
- Vascular
- Hypermobile.

PoTS can also affect the body temperature as it does with me. I also have facial flushing, often at night. I have irregular swelling and sweating of the facial tissues. In fact, as the autonomic nervous system controls organs and functions then it has the ability to impact considerably on the quality of life. I cannot say that I am any different.

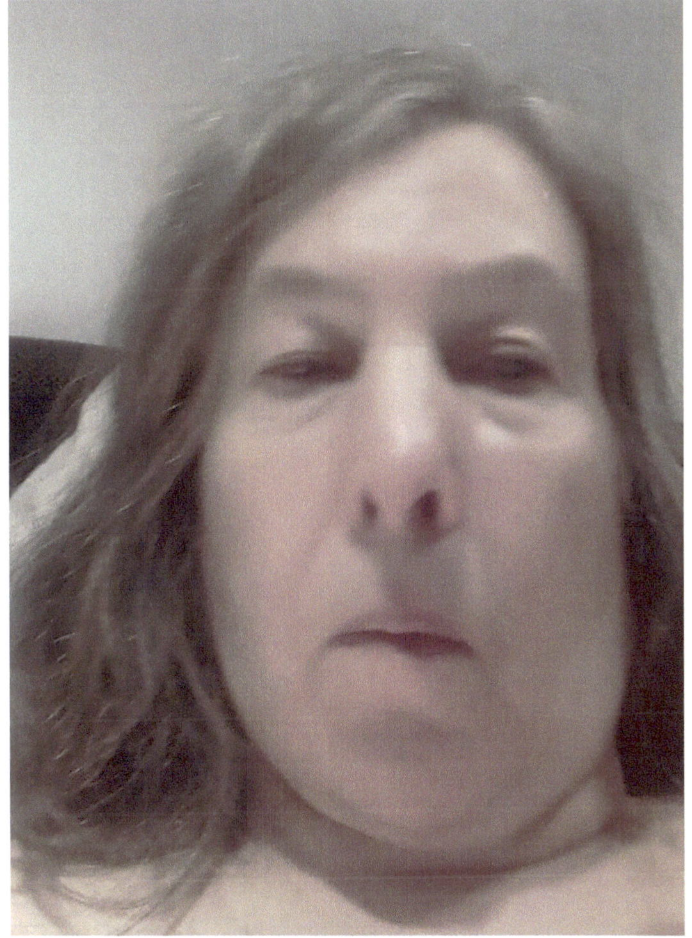

- Facial flushing, swelling of facial tissue and temperature dysregulation

I was diagnosed with MS in 1994. This is not surprising since I had Babinski's sign and subsequent MRI scans showed hundreds of lesions scattered around the parietal lobe. However, the diagnosis did not fit entirely easily given my long list of other, apparently unrelated, symptoms. There was something missing. Even the constipation- even though it is a recognised symptom of MS – did not fit easily with me that it might be MS related. I now have Gastro Oesophageal Reflux Disorder – another of those conditions which relate easily to - and are associated with - laxity of tissues. That's another bit of the missing jigsaw which is now, for me, so very nearly complete.

I did wonder why I broke a bone in my foot near the syndactic toes when they rolled under me one day. It appeared to be such a little accident which resulted in such a lot of pain. Bones are also formed from collagen so it is not surprising that they fracture easily, with little stress, when the collagen is poorly formed.

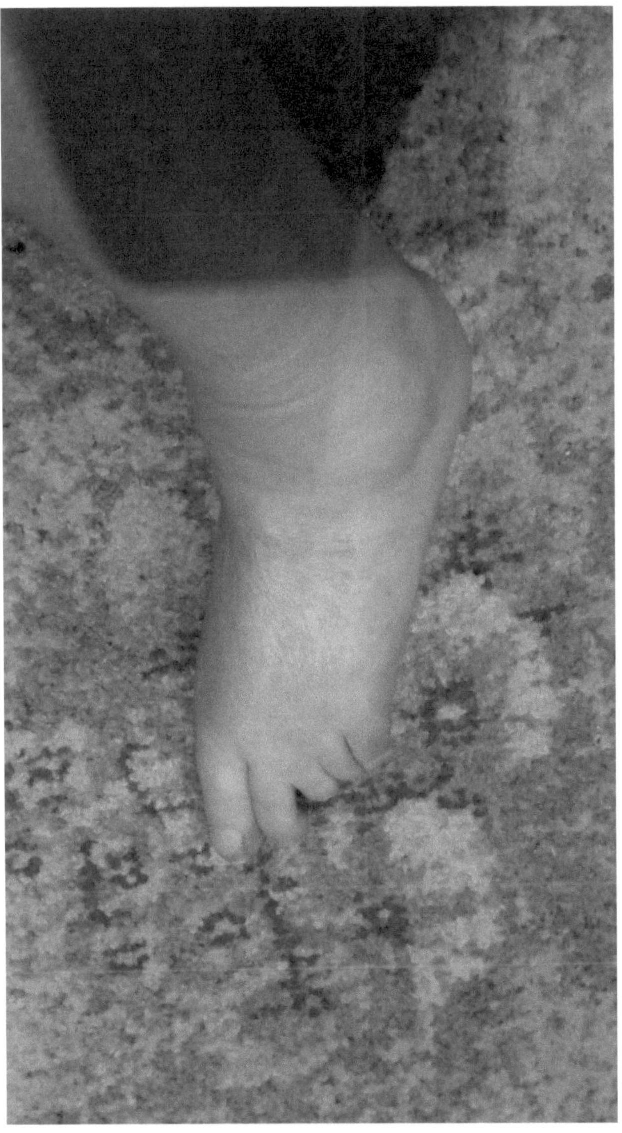

You can see why my toes roll easily underfoot can't you?

The broken bone went unnoticed and I was given steroids for another condition my former practice thought I had. Steroids are contraindicated in a connective tissue disorder as steroids will damage it even further. Steroids thin tissue and mine is already thin and poorly formed.

I have been on steroids a number of times – generally for asthma related conditions - and each time I have noticed that I have lost a little more of my function which has not returned once the course of steroids has finished.

I think it is only right to make plans for treating an individual's known conditions without steroids where these would normally be prescribed.

Where I currently am

I seem to have an adverse reaction to most medication I have ever taken for every separate symptom that I have had in my lifetime. Most of the time I just put up with the pain until it begins to get too much. Sometimes side effects of medication can be just as bad as the symptoms of EDS.

The chronic constipation is here to stay. It annoys me. It disrupts my life. It is not a subject that you share with friends over coffee, but it will, nevertheless, I be with me for the rest of my days.

I have gastroparesis with all the discomfort that this entails. The GORD wakes me up at night. There is a spasm at the bottom of my gullet and it a deep and lasting pain. I lie awake until it goes but it is always reluctant to do so.

My shoulders constantly hurt. They go into spasm and I have to catch my breath at times. I have persistent sciatica and a knee which gives way. My ankles swell should I dare walk on them. My feet 'give' when I'm walking so that I would fall over if I didn't have support.

On the 5th June 2018, I hung a shopping bag, containing one bag of sugar, over my left arm. I have been in constant and severe pain since and cannot grip with my left hand.

 On the 5th October, I travelled on a coach. On rising from the seat – where my knee had been pressing lightly against the edge of the seat, I found that I was in severe pain. I could not easily get into bed and when I did my leg kept going into spasm. I could only relieve it by getting out of bed and standing on it. This ridiculous scenario went on for two hours. It is not surprising that I am tired. I still have the pain. I am always in pain.

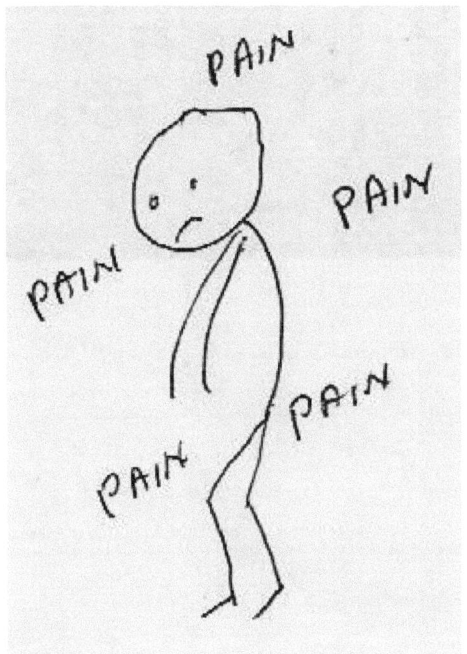

Swallowing is difficult. Again it has been there for a long time but I have not had time to acknowledge the discomfort, never mind examine it and wonder upon why it is so. Sometimes food gets lodged in the wrong place and makes me gag and, at other times, it just sits there. It is slightly uncomfortable and very inconvenient as though it has a right to be there.

I was reluctant to discuss these things with the GP. I have, after all, lived a lifetime of not being believed of living a fantasy in order to extract a small amount of benefit – a pittance – when I would rather have had the career that my intellect would have enabled me to have. It would not have been as damaging as trying to live on a pension based on a work history disrupted by illness.

My operation for the repair of the diastasis recti cost in the region of £12,000. I would have liked to have spent it on having a good retirement with my husband but I could not bend to put my shoes and socks on due to the diastasis which, as is highly probable, occurred due to my hypermobility and poor connective tissue. I had lost my independence and that was important to me.

The pain and lost opportunities are hard enough to cope with but the hardest thing to bear is the disbelief from others about the impact of the disability. I look well, after all. I do not readily show pain either.

 I do not know if it is because I have learnt that my discomfort will not be responded to or whether it is just an autistic trait. Sometimes I can walk away from the disbelieving comments and, at other times I am angry at the callousness and ignorance of people.

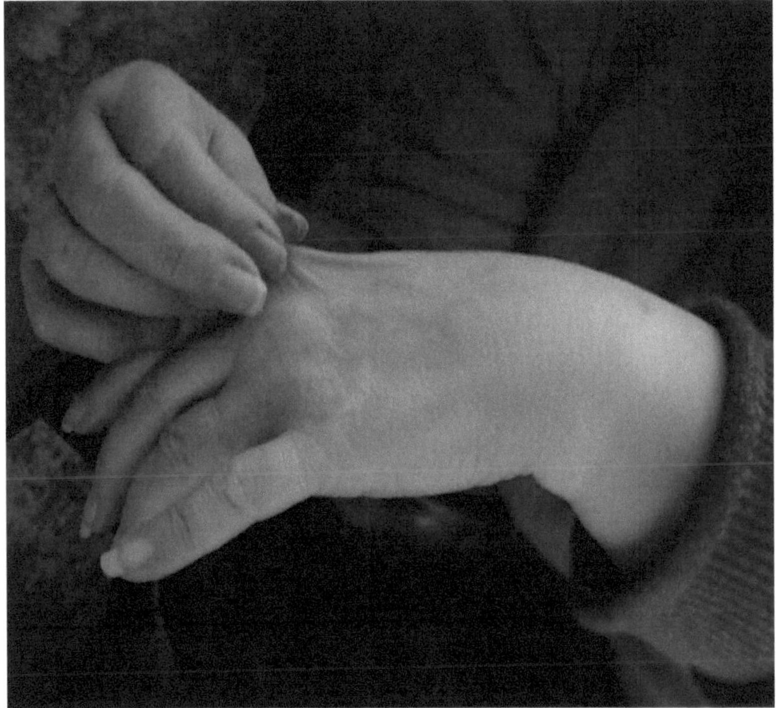

My skin is hyper-elastic but does not retain its original shape once I release it.

This next picture shows how fragile my blood vessels are.

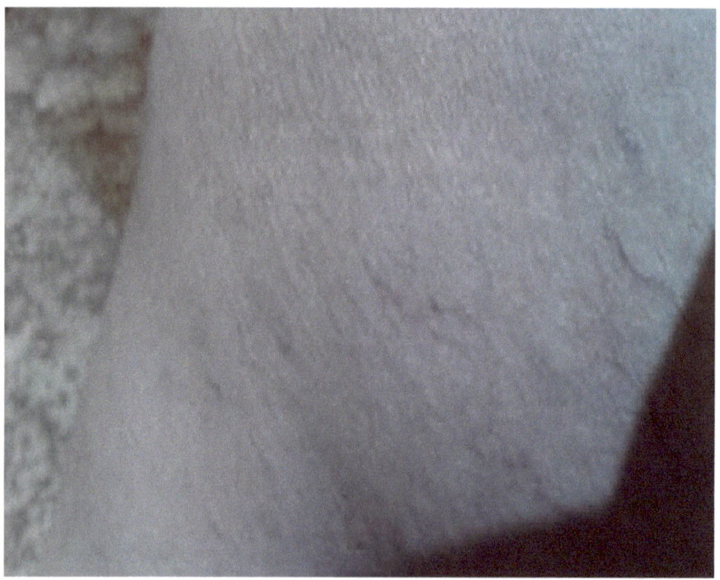

People with hypermobility syndrome tire easily. My head is still full of ideas and raring to go but after an hour of communicating verbally, I cannot make sense of anything anymore. I have to go to bed to recover. It is not surprising that I choose not to spend time in social situations. It is just too fatiguing.

Individuals with hypermobility syndrome do not heal well. When their tissue scars it has a cigarette paper like look and tends to widen but without the bleeding. Here is one of my scars which has widened since it healed.

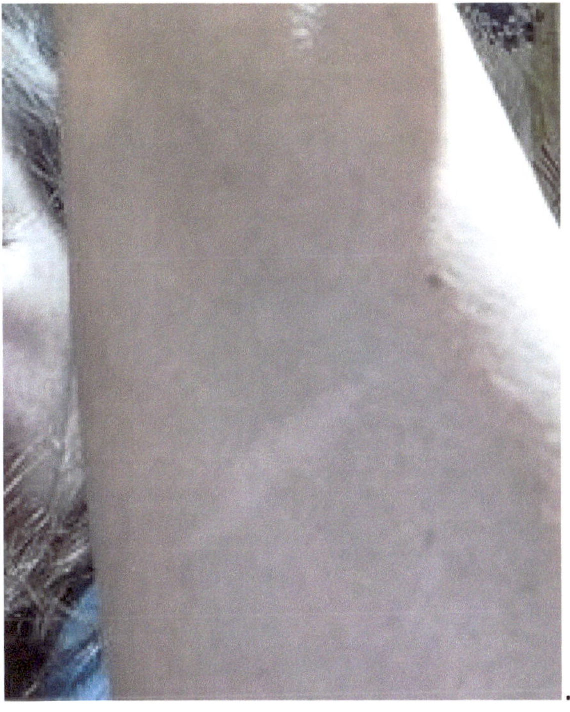

Mast cell disorders can exist alongside EDS. Mast cell are immune system cells. If the immune system is working properly then mast cells inform other cells when there is a foreign body and that they should respond to it.

However, when the immune system doesn't work properly then mast cells can cause a lot of problems with allergies, connective tissue disorders and nerve problems.

Swelling can occur. The swelling on my face is the most noticeable and also affects my ability to see.

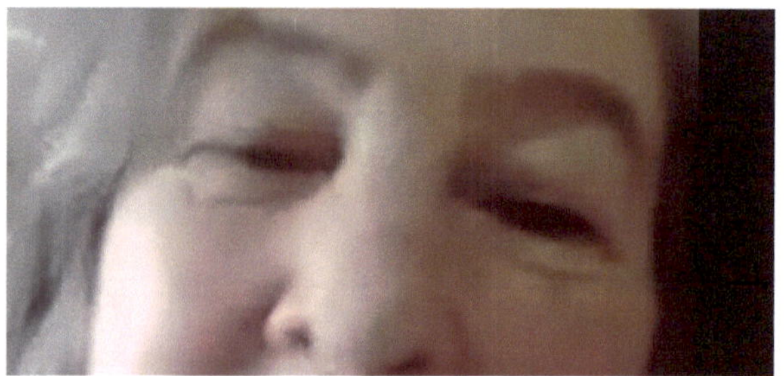

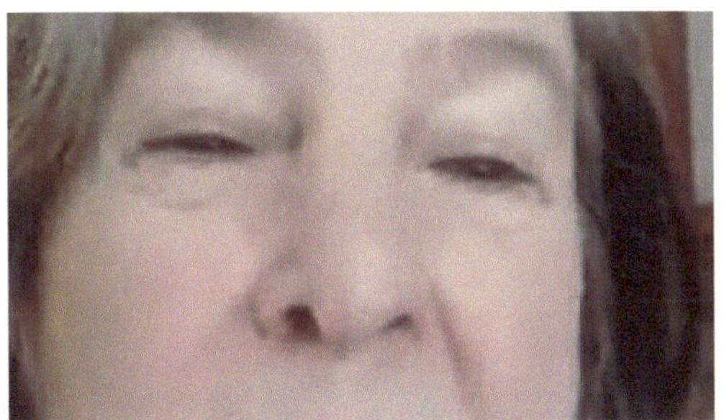

Mast Cells, Connective and Mast Cell Activation Disorder

Cells are surrounded by extra cellular matrix which is made from collagen. Collagen is important in connective tissue. Mast cells can adhere to the extra cellular matrix, which appears to alter their behaviour especially if the collagen is different as it will be in EDS.

Mast cell activation disorder (MCAD) occurs when there is an increase of mast cells. Some people with hypermobility syndrome also have MCAD suggesting an association between the conditions.

One study showed that 66% of patients with both a high heart rate when standing (PoTS) and EDS also had symptoms consistent with a form of MC activation.

Symptoms can include itching and redness and common triggers include

- Heat
- Alcohol
- Surgery
- Infection
- Stress
- Physical contact
- High body temperature

Heat and physical contact produce a similar reaction in me. I have to place cotton wool under my bra edging or I suffer intense redness and itching if I don't.

Here is an example of urticaria on my hand

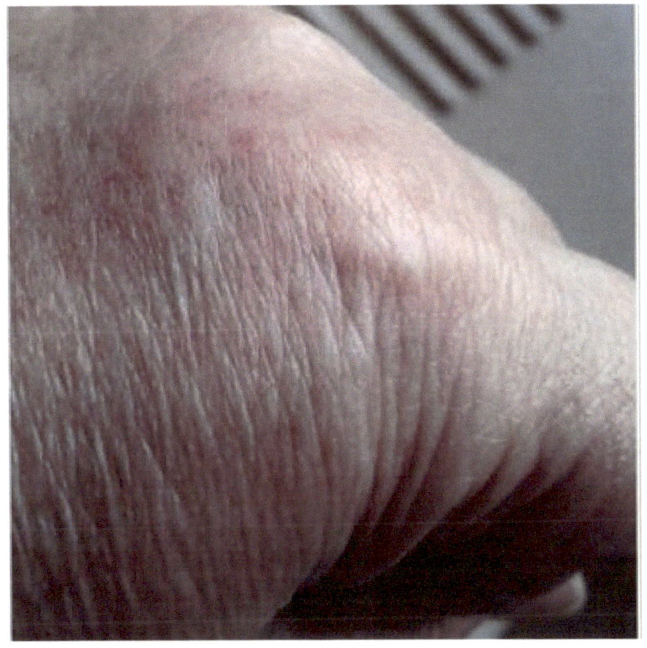

.

Treatment of MCAD

The triggers need to be identified so that they can be avoided. I know some, but not all, of mine.

Heat brings out urticaria but it is difficult to avoid in the middle of summer. I also have a pressure urticaria which means every time I walk and I exert pressure on my feet, it will cause swelling. I cannot wear tight clothing and currently, I cannot wear my wedding ring or wear a watch with a strap.

I had a reaction when I took Clarithromycin – a common antibiotic – one day. I became very tachycardic[1] and was rushed to the local hospital. It felt very peculiar as I was aware of what was going on around me but I couldn't do anything about it. This was the second dose of this antibiotic and I felt dizzy after I had taken the first dose.

 I ended up in the crash unit at the local hospital. I will not be taking Clarithromycin again.

As I have had marked swelling in my throat which occurs shortly after I have eaten – although the trigger has never been identified – I carry two Epipens around with me. I was also prescribed different types of

---

[1] Rapid heart beat

antihistamines. Some were so big that I couldn't swallow them. Some of the smaller ones caused indigestion. All of them gave me profound brain fog so that I was unable to do anything. Sometimes, you just can't win!

Commonly used medications with a mast cell activation disorder are

- Ranitidine

Ranitidine is a histamine-2 blocker. This means it reduces the amount of stomach acid made and is useful for indigestion and GORD[2].

- Sodium Cromoglycate

This is an anti-allergy medication which is useful for food allergies. It works by preventing the release of substances which would cause inflammation in the stomach

- Omlalizumab

This medication was used to reduce sensitivities to allergens

---

[2] Gastro-oesophageal Reflux Disorder – often found in connective tissue diseases due to the laxity of tissues.

- Leukotriene receptors

These are used as an add- on treatment for asthma.

Some over the counter remedies are

- Vitamin C
- Aspirin
- Cannabinoids
- Quercetin

Vitamin C helps stabilise the mast cells which cause an allergic reaction and also help decrease the amount of histamine released. It is found in good quantities in fresh fruit and vegetables. Heat kills vitamin C.

Aspirin is usually associated with causing an allergic reaction but it has been found to alleviate allergic rhinitis.

Cannabinoids have been found to alleviate seasonal allergies. There are tiny CB2 receptors on mast cells which when activated have direct anti-inflammatory effects.

Another set of receptors – the CB1 receptors, acts on bronchial nerve ending and has bronchodilating effects by acting on the bronchial nerve endings. It acts on the smooth muscle and may be beneficial in airway hyper reactivity and asthma.

Quercetin is a very useful antioxidant which has excellent anti-inflammatory properties. It is also anti-viral, anti-microbial and anti- allergy properties. These flavonoid polyphenol are most beneficial for down-regulating or suppressing inflammatory pathways. It has potent effects on immunity and inflammation caused by leukocytes and other intra cellular signals.

It certainly has mast stabilising properties.

Good sources of quercetin are capers which have the highest amount quercetin when compared with similar amounts of other quercetin containing foods. However, they are not widely eaten. Good food sources are

- Onions
- Leafy vegetable
- Broccoli
- Peppers
- Apples,

- Grapes
- Black and green tea
- Red wine
- Fruit juices

Antihistamines can be useful in that sometimes they can relieve chronic migraine headaches.

Stuffy noses respond to decongestants but some of the best decongestants are steroid based. Given the propensity of steroids to thin connective tissue when it is already fragile, it is best to keep off this type of decongestant.

Sterimar appears to work well as a decongestant and does not appear to have any unwanted side effects.

Pain

Pain can be dealt with using a wide range of analgesics including

- Ibuprofen
- Aspirin
- Paracetamol
- NSAID's (non-steroidal anti-inflammatory

However, both ibuprofen and aspirin - which are over the counter medications – are well documented as inducing anaphylaxis in susceptible people. They and NSAID's damage the delicate gut lining. NSAID'S have been found to feed damaging 'bad' bacteria and increase the risk of heart attack and stroke.

Ibuprofen and paracetamol can be taken together -, if the ibuprofen can be tolerated - and provide extra benefits when this occurs.

There are more analgesics than this but many - like those derived from opioids - have unwanted side effects such as constipation. This is already likely to be problematical in someone with a connective tissue disorder. Clearly alternative approaches to pain have to be found.

Alternative approaches to pain relief

- **Cryotherapy** – sudden intense cold reduces inflammation and numbs pain
- **Hot/cold compresses** – the alternate heat and cold reduce the inflammation around sore joints and muscles
- **Curcumin** reduces inflammation which also reduces pain
- **Some anti-histamines**, surprisingly, have the ability to reduce pain .when there has been an injury and localised infection. Some of the damaged cells release chemotactic factors which attract thousands of white cells into the area. These turn into raging phagocytes which engulf bacteria and killing them in the process. These and other cells, including mast cells, release histamine, prostaglandins and kinins. Aspirin impairs prostaglandin formation but anti-histamines prevent histamine release which also contributes to the pain and swelling of the localised inflammatory response.

It should be noted that if pain is due to localised infection then that may warrant antibiotics given that aspirin and anti-histamines have the potential to relieve pain only.

- **TENS** -Some people find this helpful but I have not. I find the pulses distracting and sometimes painful which just adds to the pain I am also feeling. Nevertheless, some people **do** find it helpful.

- **PEMF** – this is the domain of physiotherapists and is used to heal fractures and torn cartilage more quickly. Surgeons recommend it as a means to minimise soft tissue inflammation, post operatively. These machines send electromagnetic pulses through your tissue and gently stimulate anti-inflammatory compounds.

- **Vick's Vapour Rub** – an old favourite for chestiness but rubbed around joints and muscles appears to alleviate pain far better than PEMF.

- **Massage** – this helps release stress and tension that builds up in muscle tissue. Massage stimulates blood flow which allows energy to flow more freely. It improves lymph circulation which helps the body get rid of toxins

- **Home-made capsaicin cream**

Recipe for homemade Capsaicin cream:

1. Mix 3 tablespoons of cayenne powder with one cup of oil (about 200ml). You can use coconut, almond, olive oil or similar.
2. Heat the ingredients together very slowly until everything is mixed well.
3. Stir in half a cup of grated beeswax until it is completely melted.
4. Chill the mixture in the refrigerator for ten minutes or so before stirring again

- **An anti-inflammatory diet** – this includes lot of green leafy vegetables such as collards, spinach and kale/ olive oil/ nuts/ fatty fish – mackerel, tuna and sardines and fresh fruit. Pineapple, particularly, contains an inflammatory substance, known as bromelain.

The Difficulty with High Fibre Diets

For many people who have impaired gut motility such as the elderly, neuro disorder and connective tissue disorders (not a definitive list) fibre can actually make constipation worse, not better. Wholemeal grains are the worst culprits by far.

Chyme is a pulpy acidic fluid which passes from the stomach to the small intestine. It consists of gastric juices and partly digested food.

When it is fully digested, it is absorbed into the blood and 95% of the absorption of nutrients occurs in the small intestines.

Water and minerals are reabsorbed back into the blood in the colon – the large intestine – where the pH is slightly acidic.

Gastroparesis is a condition where the stomach contents empty more slowly into the small intestine than would be expected. It is considered the most common disabling motility disease. The term 'gastro' refers to the stomach and 'paresis' means weakness or paralysis.

The delayed gastric emptying that occurs in this condition may lead to secondary gastro-oesophageal reflux disease (GORD) and is occurs because the contents may back up into the oesophagus.

I can only eat small meals as I have gastroparesis and GORD. I adapted my diet to this condition without really thinking about it. This appears to be quite a common theme with me.   I have responded to perceived changes in how my body works without thinking too much about the whys and wherefores.

I have had to adopt a very soft diet; something akin to baby food. I certainly cannot eat any whole wheat grain in the form of bread or cereals without the risk of becoming impacted. When once I ate vegetables with gay abandon, I now find that my limit is two or three sprouts. Even smooth soup made with lots of vegetables can be problematical.

The diet which now suits me is the complete opposite to the one I originally used to enjoy.

I have very few vegetables in my diet. I have increased the fruit as it contains sorbitol which aids gut motility but I am not a great fan of fruit. I will eat it if it served as an accompaniment with meat.

I have to stew any meat to death. The slow cooker is very handy for this. As I generally forget it is on, the meat literally is stewed to death. This greatly softened food helps the problems caused by gastroparesis and GORD. It also helps prevent my jaw from dislocating.

 I have become quite adept at adding fruity sauces to meat. I make a batch of these in the soup-maker and freeze them for later use.   This is useful as a lot of the time I do not feel up to make anything.

I can generally only tolerate small amounts of meat. Some diets for gastroparesis suggest using only 'soft' meats such as chicken but this does limit variety.

For the most part I have had to abandon mash potato and roasts which I love. On every occasion that I eat them now I have GORD which is not just uncomfortable but also very painful. I find small amounts of white rice with the meat is acceptable.

I also keep handy free form amino acids which can be made up into a protein shake. Free form amino acids need no digestion and are absorbed immediately. Having some of these handy often takes the stress of planning meals which also take a lot of preparation.

Nevertheless, if this still isn't enough to correct the bowel problems then bowel motility agents need to be considered. It is quite likely that more than one is required. The most commonly prescribed are

Bowel Motility Agents

- Bisacodyl
- Sodium Picosulphate
- Movicol
- Resolor
- Sorbitol

 Bisacodyl is a stimulant compound and induces a bowel movement when in contact with the colon.

Sodium Picosulphate is known as a pro drug. It has no direct physiological effect on the intestine. It is however, metabolised by gut bacteria into an active compound, which is a stimulant laxative and increases peristalsis in the gut.

As this pro drug needs gut bacteria to activate it, it is unlikely to work during a course of antibiotics, or immediately after, as these kill gut bacteria so there would be no bacteria to activate the medication... As such, a substitute medication may be needed to tide the patient over during this period.

Some people say that eating yogurt would help restore the good gut bacteria. Studies are divided about whether any bacteria in yogurt could survive the hostile and acidic environment of the stomach. It is extremely acidic and its acidity helps to destroy any bacteria which is ingested.

Movicol exerts an osmotic action in the gut and this induces a laxative effect due to the increases in stool volume. This triggers colon motility via neuromuscular pathways.

Resolor is a prescription only medication which is generally prescribed for women since that is the group which studies were undertaken on. It increases gut motility in a much more 'normal' way than some of the more powerful gut motility agents. It does not appear to have any unwanted side effects.

Sorbitol – this is a sweet tasting crystalline compound found in some fruit which helps to accelerate small bowel transit. It is used in a lot of foods prepared for diabetic use.

Fruits which are good sources of sorbitol are:

Apples, pears, cherries, plums, prunes, dates, fruits with seeds such as apricots and, nectarines. Some people develop a sensitivity to sorbitol so, like anything else, you have to build up a bespoke range of medication which meet your needs. This will differ for everyone.

Some bowel medicines are probably not suited to gastroparesis if prescribed alone. Lactulose, for example, increases the amount of water in the stools.

This softens them and makes them easier to pass but if gut motility is affected as is so often the case, then the build-up of stool, can be very uncomfortable and a stimulating medication needs to be added.

Travelling on holiday

Going on holiday takes a lot of preparation. I have to take every type of medication to cover every symptom that may occur. This includes

- Pain medications
- Pain gel
- Medication to relieve GORD
- Three types of bowel medication
- Diuretic
- Medication for muscle spasms
- Ointment in case of rosacea flare up
- Ointment for application to scalp for psoriasis flare up
- 2 X Epipens
- Antihistamines
- Bandages for when joints get too painful
- Splints for walking to try and reduce sprains
- Ointment in case chazalion flares up
- Soap less cleanser as I have sensitive skin
- Betnovate for skin flare ups

- Inhaler
- Rescue antibiotics
- Sterimar
- Soap less cleanser
- Pads

This is not a definitive list.

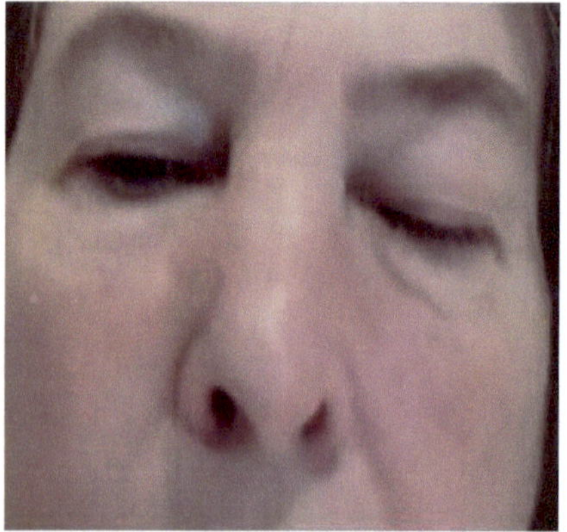

This is how the chazalion affects my eye.

As I cannot pull a suitcase, it is left to my husband to be responsible for the luggage. To aid this I only pack a small suitcase., By the time that I have the items list above, in the suitcase there is just enough room for a change of underwear, a couple of t shirts and an extra pair of trousers.

Eating -

Eating is a problem for me and not just because I have to cope with the gastroparesis and GORD which I have already mentioned. I changed the way I ate, in my twenties, when I had months of temporal mandibular disorder – not that I knew what it was them. The difficulties I had with this condition went on for months. I stopped eating anything crunchy and had to hold the side of my face when I was chewing. I could only eat small amounts of soft food at a time.

I have adapted over the years although food preparation takes a lot longer. I can't just throw anything together. I was once asked by someone who had come to assess me how I ate steak. This was in response to my honest statement that I ate using only one hand. I am quite adept at this because I 'cut' my food with the side of a fork. That's because I eat only soft food.

I informed the assessor that I did not eat steak but he insisted that I did. He demanded to know how I would cut it up and eat it and I stated quite truthfully that I wouldn't eat steak but if I was forced to then I would have to tear tiny pieces up with my hands.

His face was a picture of disbelief which just goes to show that assessors really don't understand disability and shouldn't be assessing for the effects of it

The swallowing problems probably arrived around the same time.   Food gets stuck in my oesophagus. Wholemeal bread and potatoes are the main culprit so any bread I have is lubricated well with butter and I never eat without having a cup of tea at my side to help wash it down.

It is a challenge eating out but this is something that we have to do sometimes when my husband and I are too tired to make something. Sometimes the simple act of having someone else make a sandwich is appreciated more than is realised. I make sandwiches with the softer white bread. I still have to eat it in very small bites but at least it does not get lodged as easily as wholemeal bread and cereals do.

Of course, this all takes time and money. I have simply come to understand that people either do not understand the price of disability, or the time involved in attending to it, or would prefer not to think about it so that they don't have to address the issue.   This takes me neatly onto the next subject which is the high cost of having a disability; that is, disability related expenses.

Disability related expenses

Every disability will bring with it, its own set of expenses. These will be dynamic because most conditions are. They symptoms come and go when you least expect it. Some symptoms disappear permanently but are replaced by others. Some symptoms intensify.

The disability related expenses I have cannot be quantified but they include

- Soap less wash – I have flare ups of psoriasis and rosacea and my skin appears very sensitive to a lot of things.
- Heating – I can't regulate my body temperature
- Laptop (for communication)
- Bandages
- OTC medicines not obtained from GP
- Breakdown cover
- Specialist shoes in more than one size to account for swelling
- Travel insurance – horrendous

- Kitchen gadgets to accommodate for weak wrists/ liquidise food
- Cotton and woollen clothing – much more expensive than off the peg clothing I would otherwise buy from Primark.
- Samsung Tablet to take photos of disability as it arises
- Petrol costs – I cannot access the bus otherwise I would use my free bus pass. The cost of petrol for hospital appointments and just generally getting around far exceeds that which is allowed for disability
- Disability rooms in hotels when we visit relatives.
- Costs of proving I have a disability to agencies who know I have one! For example, I need to purchase my medical notes for ATOS and send ones supporting my disabilities even though they contact my GP/consultants to check my assertions...
- Extra washing and washing powder
- Ear plugs – my hearing is sensitive.
- Special pens – I can only hold one type comfortably.

- Cost of making kitchen adapted to suit my needs
- Cost of cleaner as I cannot push the vacuum cleaner any more
- Gardener – I cannot garden anymore: I constantly sprain my joints when I do so.
- Cost of domestic help. I cannot hang washing up nor pick up the iron. Neither can I sit for more than about ten minutes without being propped up if I am to avoid being in pain
- Cost of someone to adapt clothing to accommodate swelling and also avoid physical pressure
- Cost of someone to help me carry shopping.
- Costs of travel to hospital and, if waiting for a long time, costs for food and drink to sustain over the time there. Hospital food is especially expensive.
- Cost of eating out when too tired to cook.
- Batteries for kitchen gadgets like tin openers.
- Cost of cotton wool as I have to line around the edges of clothing in order to avoid an urticarial flare up.
- Insoles. I was allowed one pair of insoles by our local hospital's orthotics department but they

were very hard and hurt my feet so much that I could not wear them. I eventually saw a private podiatrist and obtained some bespoke ones from her. They were not cheap but at least I could wear them.

What I would have liked the medical profession to have done

I am sixty five now and had lived with constant pain all my life. It is not a figment of my imagination, the medics have seen my swollen joints and seen the disability it causes. I have turned up numerous times in A&E or to see consultants to present with yet another joint injury or back pain. The excessive pronation of my ankles and hypermobility of joints are in evidence yet no-one has ever suggested a connective tissue disorder.

Apparently, it takes on average nineteen years to diagnose a connective tissue disorder such as EDS. That's nineteen years of being on the end of pain and judgemental others, of not being able to put a name to something which would legitimise it and make you less likely to be viewed with suspicion as someone who is trying to defraud the public purse. In my case it has taken a lifetime. I am sixty five!

To be fair if someone had asked me if I had hypermobile joints I would have probably said, 'No!'

I have lived with my knees and my toes and my pain all my life. They are my normality. This is why I depended on other people to do the thinking for me. It would not have been too much trouble to have produced a chart and asked have you ever sprained, dislocated or had pain in this joint. I would have been able to answer yes to every one of my joints being affected with tendonitis by the time I was in my mid-twenties.

Perhaps, while we are sitting in the Practice waiting room, there could be a highly visible chart asking if we could ever touch our wrist with the thumb on the same side. If so, please discuss with your GP.

Sometimes we need permission to do this. We feel that it is too much trouble to discuss that we bruise easily or heal badly or are always in pain. Why should anyone believe us when we say that opening a drawer can result in us spraining our wrist? I have certainly had doubt cast on my assertions that this has been the case, in the long distant past. I learned to keep quiet a long time ago when a physio I attended suggested I was making my pain up as a way to have physical contact with another person. I do wonder, at times, why people with such muddled heads go into the caring professions.

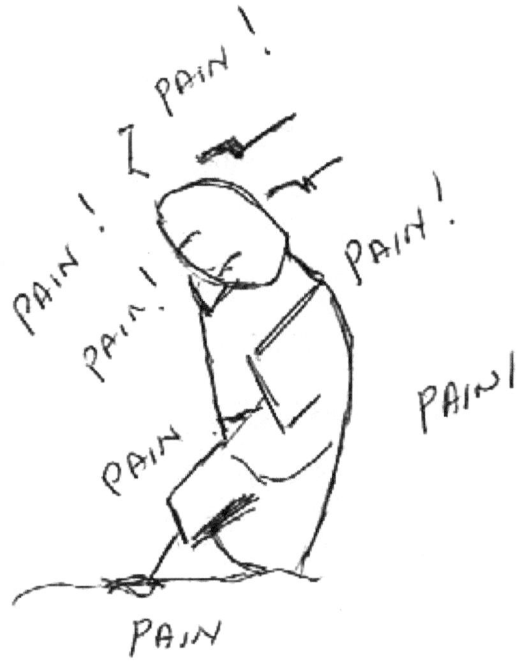
PAIN !
PAIN !
PAIN !
PAIN !
PAIN !
PAIN !
PAIN
PAIN
PAIN

Social services – I have never known anyone in this profession who understands disability, the expense of disability and the impact it has on your life including the financial and academic implications.

Social workers, I have found, while stating that they haveno medical training at all appear to be making judgements on medical issues.

They see only a snapshot of people's lives as do assessors who pop up once every three years to chop, shape and make a decision on somebody's life of whom they know nothing about.

I had to cancel three appointments - through ill-health - to assess my disability. On the fourth occasion I was able to keep the appointment as I was well enough. Decisions were then based entirely on my ability to do tasks on the day I was well to be involved in a meeting even though that only represented 25% of the time when I actually was well enough to do so.

Connective tissue disorders are often invisible. Fatigue and pain aren't always apparent especially with the older generation who soldier on regardless - or for people like me who have no choice in the matter anyway.

And, of course, the fact that our pain has not been given a legitimate name does not make it any less painful or less of a disruption to our lives. It still affects our ability to work and has a knock on effect on our pension. Make no mistake!

Nevertheless, until it is given a name it has little legitimacy in the eyes of many professionals. We become victims of a condition we did not want in the first place.

It would be an understatement to say that I now don't trust any officer from the local authority.

I am sure that somewhere will be their observation that I have 'trust issues' – a common form of a social workers repertoire of professional jargon. I know this because I used to lecture in social care issues to student social workers and decried the use of professional jargon then. It actually prevents the social worker from thinking objectively and creatively, in their responses, to some of the problems that their clients face, when they rely heavily on pre-rehearsed phrases.

It is a little arrogant, however, on their part to believe that they should be wholly trusted when they have repeatedly failed to implement the Care Act in a professional and objective way. If that was the case then I could legitimately be labelled as having a personality disorder.

Further, it is my observation that any assistance offered is based not on need, but on personalities.

To illustrate this, when my husband and I first approached our local authority for some assistance which, at the time, would only have been temporary, the Deputy Team Manager wrote in her notes that we were an 'eccentric' couple.

My husband has worked hard all his life as an architect, landscape architect and university lecturer for some very prestigious and famous names while taking care of his very ill mother. He is the glue that binds a community together. He spent over a year popping in daily to see a gentleman with dementia and has given his professional services free to individuals and community groups so that they can continue their good work.

If eccentricity measures kindness and integrity then my husband has it in bucket loads. However, it is clear that the deputy team manager did not mean it as a positive comment. While my husband has since received an apology, I am still waiting for mine.

What helps?

It helps having a good GP practice and I am fortunate that I do have that. The five main things you require from your GP practice is

- A high level of professional competence
- A 'can do' approach
- The willingness to listen and act when necessary
- Someone you can get on with
- Approachable receptionists

So 5/5 here although it has taken me 65 years to find such a practice. In fact the only drawback is that I live in a village. I can't drive and there is only one bus going in that direction, hourly, I cannot get there unless there is someone available to take me. Planning an appointment is, therefore, a bit of a marathon task at the best of times.

Arm yourself with the relevant literature

If you do have a firm diagnosis of a troublesome medical condition such as a connective tissue disorder, then it helps to be armed with leaflets and website addresses for the non-medical people who may be involved in your care. I have found that while these professionals may say they understand complex physical and mental needs, I have found that this just isn't true and sadly, they lump conditions (not disorders) like autistic spectrum difference and ADHD together and file them under mental health conditions instead of celebrating the unique contribution each group can play in society. If there is a 'mental' health condition attached it is highly likely a reaction to the way that the mainstream treats those who are different.

The autistics logic is unrivalled and research has shown that those with ADHD are gifted with entrepreneurship.

Take photographs of the signs of your illness.

I found that my Samsung tablet was one of my best allies, documenting the signs of my unpredictable condition and silencing the disbelievers. It gave my pain legitimacy. It made me feel more secure. It has helped me illustrate this book.

Learn to develop a tough skin.

With any chronic medical condition, it is living in a fantasy land to believe that every professional involved in your condition will be able or willing to respond appropriately. Some of the reasons are:-

- Personality differences
- Ignorance of a condition and an unwillingness to learn about it
- Lack of empathy from the professional
- Lack of money in the system to accommodate legitimate needs

Actually, the latter reason should not apply as the law currently states that local authorities should not deny people adequate care on the basis that there is no money in the system. The law states that the local authority should use their reserves –this is a piece of legislation which my own particular local authority don't appear to be aware of.

However, down the road, is Wakefield local authority. It is responsive and caring. I have been privileged to have met many clients of Wakefield local authority and **not one** has had a bad word to say this authority. Indeed, they sing its praises. I have to ask myself if one local authority can manage to fulfil its responsibilities why can't mine?

So, it helps to be armed with some knowledge of the law so that when mistruths about what is available, are fed to you, you are able to counteract them.

Understand the local authority complaint's process and don't be shy of asking for it. The complaint's process should be implemented as a way for the organisation to look at issues which the client finds unfair.   However, in every case but one, my observation is that organisations use the allotted time of eight weeks for the process, to try and find a loophole so that they don't have to address legitimate issues.

This happens so often now that I expect it and build in that time before I will receive a final response and can then take it to the next independent stage

Most organisations bank on you giving up well before then. You have to be a particularly determined person to go through the whole process. Consider it a learning experience and don't expect any justice until you get to the independent stage but make sure that you do take your complaint that far.

It is helpful to be in touch with organisations who can support you on your journey whether these are organisations which deal specifically with your condition or organisations which can help you obtain your human rights. It is always better to be prepared.

Local authorities do have to provide an independent advocate for people who are vulnerable. In my own case my 'vulnerability' is my inability to be able to cognitively process and produce a verbal response in the time allotted in a meeting. I can well fight my corner on paper!

Under Section 36 of the Data Protection Act, clients are allowed to record meetings – with or without an individual's permission or knowledge – for domestic purposes. Organisations do not enjoy the same rights as they do have to inform you if they are recording a conversation. My advice is to **always record** meetings. I have no objections to the other side doing so either. It is a necessary safeguard.

Become an expert patient

This really is a responsibility which a patient should undertake. It is not unusual for a patient to turn up at hospital or a new GP practice to find that they know little of a particularly rare disorder. Often patients become the experts in their conditions and can work together with medical professionals to improve their conditions.

Find something that you can do well

I write! I write about a great many things on many different subjects – on social justice, health and magical children's stories.

I have a blog which has a readership in the US, Canada, Colombia, Australia and New Zealand among others. Social issues are an important part of my life – my first modules with the university were on social issues before I moved onto educational and finally medical issues.

I like to uncover the injustices in society and give them an airing. I am not concerned with the ordinary person who makes a mistake now and again. Everyone makes mistakes. I do too! I am concerned about the systemic abuse which is so often found to go hand in hand with local authorities and other large organisations.

This gives me an outlet for some of my abilities when other avenues are closed due to physical limitations.

It is true that people need to feel valued and have a sense that they are contributing to society somehow. Chronic pain can limit choices but it still allows some. This is what needs to be explored, reflected upon and put into practise for the sake of your own mental health.

Some people join and contribute to charities dealing with their own particular conditions and get a great sense of satisfaction out of doing so.

 If you haven't already done it, find something that you do well and enjoy doing. It will make a huge difference to your life.

Finally

The road to finding a legitimate label for chronic disease is a long and often lonely one. It is journey one shouldn't walk by oneself but that would not adequately describe the reality of the situation.

Along the way one would hope to find helpers but, too often willingness is not entwined with competence or understanding leaving the sojourner feeling even more isolated.

Then there are those whose sole job is to pour judgement and disbelief and denial on one's experience. There are really only few remedies for this type of injustice and these are

- to walk away
- to challenge the misperceptions

The former may be easier but is unlikely, in contrast to the second option, to make lasting changes.

Good Luck – whichever way you choose to go!

Useful Information

Ehlers Danlos Support UK

https://www.ehlers-danlos.org/

The Beighton Score

The Beighton Score is an indicator of widespread hypermobility but a high score, by itself, is not necessarily an indicator that someone has hypermobility syndrome. There needs to be other signs and symptoms present.

A low score does not necessarily mean that hypermobility is not present. Not every joint is counted in the Beighton scale. For example dislocation of the jaw, shoulders and feet are not counted in the Beighton hypermobility score.

The Beighton Score is calculated as follows

- One point is you can place your palms flat on the ground while your legs are straight
- One point for each elbow which bends backwards
- One point for each knee that bends backwards
- One point for each thumb which can bend and touch the wrist on the same side
- One point for each little finger that bends backwards beyond 90^0

A score of 4 point raises the concern that a generalised hypermobility might be present.

Hypermobility Questionnaire.

An answer to any two questions on the hypermobility questionnaire gives a high likelihood of the presence of hypermobility. However, this does not mean that the individual has Hypermobility Syndrome.

- Can you now- or could you ever – place your hands flat on the floor without bending your knees?
- Can you now – or could you ever – bend your thumb to touch your forearm?
- As a child did you amuse your friends by contorting your body into unusual shapes or could you do the splits?
- As a child or teenager did your shoulder or kneecap dislocate on more than one occasion?
- Do you consider yourself double-jointed?

https://quintessentiallylynne.weebly.com/about.html

www.ingramcontent.com/pod-product-compliance
Lightning Source LLC
Chambersburg PA
CBHW040224240726
48664CB00001B/4